Legal & Disclaimer

Contents

Introduction

With aging comes a celebration of many things – sweet grandchildren clinging on to grandpa and grandma, asking endless questions about the days gone by; a sense of accomplishment for a life well-lived, and wisdom that is being passed on to children and their offspring. However, with aging also comes some unwelcome visitors - sleeplessness, weakness, occasional to regular pains, and, the hardest of all to live with and accept, sicknesses or illnesses that deprive us of the liberty to be what we want to be and go where we want to go. Many older people have these aforementioned issues, in tandem with being unable to enjoy the same food and drinks and other little indulgences that they used to savor in the past. The confinement and the restrictions imposed by these diseases are more debilitating than the actual threats. So, we sigh. Don't we deserve some relief? Some rest? Some joys of life even during these sunset years?

There's good news! Being advanced in years doesn't have to be so confining. Just because you are a senior doesn't mean you always have to be in a restrictive environment, characterized by endless pains and aches. You can be free, or at the very least, be able to eliminate these pains, go on with your senior years and enjoy life as everyone should.

Unfortunately, not many seniors are aware of the secrets, and these are what you are going to uncover in this specially made eBook for the aging individuals. You will find out that you can live each day with fewer body pains and a greater pain tolerance, and at times, experience the relief that you have always longed to have.

I am so glad you've availed of this material; this is a treasure, your guide towards a better quality of life at this stage of your existence. As you experience these happy days, you will find more time to enjoy life at its best, doing the things you love, being with family and so much more.

In this eBook, I have provided proven Traditional Healing Methods that are waiting to be tapped into by you. In the pages of Chapter 1, you will find out what these are and what are involved, and how to take advantage of them for your own benefit. Furthermore, in Chapter 2 you will be exposed to all of the information that you need to know about Essential Oils and how they can make your life significantly better. You will discover that you have deprived yourself a lot by not knowing these secrets.

There are other sections written just for you. Chapter 3 tells you the reasons Why Every Home Should Have Essential Oils, and you'll be glad you have them. This will be followed by Chapter 4 where you will learn the secrets of Achieving a Better Life Through Essential Oils.

Finally, this eBook gives you all the things you need to know on How to Prepare Essential Oils for a Healthier Living.

Let your journey to a better and healthier living begin with this outstanding material on Essential Oils, details that you have never before encountered.

Chapter 1- Traditional Healing Methods Waiting to be Discovered

You can be healthier, and you can definitely feel better with the traditional healing procedures and- methods that have long been used prior to the discovery of conventional medicines. I am referring to aromatherapy.

Long before humankind was introduced to pills, tablets, injections, and other forms of modern medicines, people of all civilizations – from China to Africa, from the ancient Near East to the Western world – treated their sick using what was available around them. It was natural for them to resort to natural remedies such as herbs, which contained essential oils whose properties were responsible for achieving relief and healing.

Now, even with the tremendous advancement in our world today, people find that wellness can be achieved through the traditional way, and they are right. Countless individuals across the globe have realized that good health and healing can be achieved through the natural means. This is through the use of essential oils in a method called aromatherapy.

What is so amazing about aromatherapy is that it is effective in so many ways and the known side effects are negligible or minimal compared to those wrought by modern medicine. This is why people from all walks of life – from the young and the not –so-young resort to scents for wellness. Hollywood celebrities are known users of aromatherapy. Kirsten Dunst, for instance, is reported to have been using chamomile, lavender, and melissa to address her sleeping problems. In addition, she is said to be into geranium, verbena, thyme and orange oils to deal with bouts of depressive mood states. Both insomnia and depression are very common among the elderly and as others have proven the effectiveness of aromatherapy, it's high time you consider this ancient method now that you are in your advanced years. What I'm saying is that, if younger, healthier individuals find it necessary to use essential oils, all the more reason the elderly should!

Understanding Aromatherapy

As the term implies, aromatherapy is about healing, hence the word therapy. Healing or therapy is achieved by the use of scents or fragrances, usually from essential oils, which are known for their aromatic properties; hence the word aroma. In short, aromatherapy is the use of essential oils and aromatic properties of fruits, flowers, and other plants to make a person revitalized, relieved, and healed.

When we talk about healing, we mean holistic healing, and this includes physical, mental, and emotional wellness.

For some people, their challenge is more of a physical nature while others are battling emotional or mental problems. Still, others may have a combination of all three general wellness issues. Aromatherapy brings healing and dramatic relief to the physical pains, emotional struggles, and mental issues.

Dementia, insomnia, depression, circulation issues, arthritis and body pains have been relieved by the use of essential oils via aromatherapy. Even respiratory illnesses and skin degeneration, which are associated with aging, are cured with the use of essential oils or aromatherapy. Another benefit of aromatherapy is its calming, anxiolytic effect. With these benefits in mind, it would appear essential that elderly people whom are suffering at least give essential oils a shot, as they are empirically proven to help in a myriad of ways!

Administering Aromatherapy

There are a variety of ways to receive aromatherapy or administer it to others, such as the elderly. Some of these methods are through baths or showers, massages, inhaling oils, and candles, topical and sublingual use- Although most of the oils have pleasant scent, other fragrances may be found too strong by some who are particularly sensitive. Be sure you let your elderly loved one smell the scent first before using the oil.

Bath or Showers. For an elderly to experience relief from various body pains such as arthritis, some essential oils can be used during baths or showers. Administration via baths and showers are a good way to relax the bodies of the elderly. Water, usually warm or hot, is mixed with carrier oil and essential oils. You may also add a small amount of shampoo or shower gel. Use mild shampoos and gels only as aging people develop sensitive skin over time. Proper dilution rate is discussed in Chapter 4.

Massages. Before administering massages, make sure you consult a health expert and ask their opinions. Some essential oils may not be suitable, so be sure to ask the recipient of the therapy questions regarding their needs and desires or do a little safe experimenting. Frequently ask if the scents are helping or not, or instruct your loved one to tell you when a particular oil has ceased to be beneficial. Also talk to the person and inquire as to if the therapy is helping them with their prominent issues. In some cases, select oils cause some reactions with medicines or illnesses.

Aging people have sensitive skin and can be bruised easily, so make sure massage treatment is gentle. Note, too, that some essential oils can cause skin irritations especially to the seniors because of their thin epidermis. Citrus-based oils such as lemon and oranges, are a bit strong and can cause irritations, the same goes for basil, peppermint, wintergreen, cinnamon, pine, and ginger. Further, some oils can cause changes in skin color so be on the lookout for these.

Massages can take many forms. They can be done on the entire body or localized portions only. Essential oils can be used for hand and arm massage for example.

Other areas where massages may be needed are the back, legs, shoulders, and head. Again, don't forget to ask your loved one if they like the scent of a particular oil that you intend to use. If not, try other alternatives.

In massaging, you may combine unscented lotion with some essential oils such as peppermint or lavender. Citrus is also a good oil to mix with any unscented lotion.

Inhaling Oils. Aside from baths and massages, inhaling the scent of essential oils also treats various conditions. When people, especially seniors, inhale the fragrance of these oils, they begin to relax and experience a happy feeling. To inhale the scent, simply put a few drops on the palm and then rub in the oil, or use a couple of drops on a paper strip and then inhale. Cotton swabs are also used for inhaling essential oil scents and can be placed near the person who needs them such as near or under their pillow.

Another effective way of inhaling the therapeutic scents of essential oils is through the use of diffusers or humidifiers. Diffusers come in different forms and people have been creative in this area. They diffuse the scent through an electric diffuser or by placing a wooden stick in a vase filled with essential oil.

Candles. Aromatherapy can be enjoyed anywhere anytime by the use of candles. Choose your own candles and add a few drops of essential oils to them. The scents of essential oils can have various effects. They can calm the mind and relax tense and agitated individuals. The fragrance can also enhance positive feelings, mental alertness, and memory. Place the candles in glass jars or electric cup warmers which are quite affordable.

Chapter 2- What You Need to Know About Essential Oils

We believe in the saying that "Knowledge is power" and that doom comes from ignorance or lack of knowledge. Unfortunately, many of us including seniors are unnecessarily suffering from body pains and aches because they are unaware of available natural solutions. I am talking about essential oils. These oils can spell the difference in the way we live our lives. For seniors, these could be the answers you have been looking for.

What are essential oils? According to the International Organization for Standardization (ISO) essential oils are products "made by distillation with either water or steam or by mechanical processing...by dry distillation of natural materials"(NAHA, 2016). An essential oil is considered true or pure if it is extracted using physical means via distillation and expression, which is also known as cold pressing. Maceration is another method used in isolating essential oils from plants and is often used for obtaining oils from onion, garlic, wintergreen, and bitter almond.

So for you to enjoy these solutions, you first need to know what these essential oils are, where they are sourced, how they are produced or made, etc. Below is a list of Essential Oils indicating their common or popular names and their botanical or Latin names. Also provided in this chapter are the general benefits or uses of these oils.

Common or Popular Names of Essential Oils	Latin or Botanical Names of Essential Oils
Angelica	Angelica archangelica
Anise	Pimpinella anisum
Balsam Fir	Abies balsamea
Basil	Ocimum basilicum
Bergamot	Citrus bergamia
Birch (Yellow Birch)	Betula alleghaniensis

Black Pepper	Piper nigrum
Blue Cypress	Callitrus intratropica
Cajeput	Melaleuca leucadendra
Canadian Red Cedar	Thuja plicata
Cardamom	Elettaria cardamomum
Carrot	Daucua carota
Cassia	Cinnamomum cassia
Cedar, Canadian Red	Thuja plicata
Cedar, Western Red	Thuja plicata
Cedar Leaf (Thuja)	Thuja occidentalis
Cedarwood	Cedrus atlantica
Chamomile, German (Blue)	Matricaria recutita
Chamomile, Mixta	Chamaemelum mixtum
Chamomile, Roman	Chamaemelum nobile
Cinnamon Bark	Cinnamomum verum
Cistus (Labdanum)	Cistus ladanifer
Citronella	Cymbopogon nardus
Clary Sage	Salvia sclarea
Clove	Syzygium aromaticum
Coriander	Coriandrum savitum L.
Cumin	Cuminum cyminum
Cypress	Cupressus sempervirens

Cypress, Blue	Callitris intratropica
Davana	Artemisia pallens
Dill	Anethum graveolens
Douglass Fir	Pseudotsuga menziesii
Elemi	Canarium luzonicum
Eucalyptus	Eucalyptus globulus
Eucalyptus Citriodora	Eucalyptus citriodora
Eucalyptus Dives	Eucalyptus dives
Eucalyptus Polybractea	Eucalyptus polybractea
Eucalyptus Radiata	Eucalyptus radiata
Fennel	Foeniculum vulgare
Fir (Silver Fir or Fir Needle)	Abies alba
Fir, Balsam (Canadian Balsam)	Abies balsamea
Fir, Douglas	Pseudotsuga menziesii
Fir, Idaho Balsam	Abies grandis
Fir, White	Abies grandis
Fleabane	Conyza canadensis
Frankincense (Olibanum)	Boswellia carterii
Galbanum	Ferula gummosa
Geranium	Pelargonium graveolens
German Chamomile	Matriacaria recututa
Ginger	Zingiber officinale

Goldenrod	Solidago Canadensis
Grapefruit	Citrus x paradisi
Helichrysum	Helichrysum italicum
Hyssop	Hyssopus officinalis
Idaho Balsam Fir	Abies grandis
Idaho Tansy	Tanacetum vulgare
Jasmine	Jasminum officinale
Juniper	Juniperus osteosperma and/or J. scoluporum
Laurel (Bay or Bay Laurel)	Laurus nobilis
Lavandin	Lavandula x hybrida
Lavender	Lavandula angustifolia, CT Linalol
Ledum	Ledum groenlandicum
Lemon	Citrus limon
Lemongrass	Cymbopogon flexuosus
Lime	Citrus aurantifolia
Mandarin	Citrus reticulata
Marjoram	Origanum majorana
Melaleuca (Tea Tree)	Melaleuca alternifolia
Melaleca Ericifolia (Rosalina)	Melaleuca ericifolia
Melaleuca Leucadendron	Melaleuca Leucadendra
Melaleuca Quinquenervia	Melaleuca quinquenervia

(Niaouli)	
Melissa (Lemon Balm)	Melissa officinalis
Mountain Savory (Winter Savory)	Satureja montana
Mugwort	Artemisia vulgaris
Myrrh	Commiphora myrrha
Myrtle	Myrtus communis
Neroli (Orange Blossom)	Citrus aurantium bigaradia
Niaouli	Melaleuca quinquenervia
Nutmeg	Myristica fragrans
Onycha (Benzoin)	Styrax benzoin
Orange	Citrus sinensis
Oregano	Origanum vulgare, CT Carvacrol
Palmarosa	Cymbopogon martinii
Patchouly	Pogostemon cablin
Pepper, Black	Piper nigrum
Peppermint	Mentha piperita
Petitgrain	Citrus aurantium
Pine (Scotch Pine)	Pinus sylvestris
Ravensara	Ravensara aromatica
Roman chamomile	Chamaemelum nobile
Rosalina	Melaleuca ericifolia
Rose (Bulgarian Rose)	Rosa damascena

Rosehip	Rosa canina
Rosemary Cineol	Rosmarinus officinalis, CT 1,8 Cineol
Rosemary Verbenon	Rosmarinus officinalis, CT Verbenon
Rosewood	Aniba rosaeodora
Sage	Salvia officinalis
Sandalwood	Santalum album
Spearmint	Mentha spicata, CT Carvone
Spikenard	Nardostachys jatamansi
Spruce (Black Spruce)	Picea mariana
Tamanu	Calophyllum inophyllum
Tangerine	Citrus nobilis
Tansy, Blue	Tanacetum annum
Tansy, Idaho	Tanacetum vulgare
Tarragon	Artemisia dracunculus
Thyme	Thymus vulgaris, CT Thymol
Thyme Linalol	Thymus vulgaris, CT Linalol
Tsuga (Hemlock)	Tsuga canadensis
Valerian	Valeriana officinalis
Vetiver	**Vetiveria zizanoides**
Vitex	**Vitex negundo**
Western Red Cedar	Thuja plicata

White Fir	Abies grandis
White Lotus	Nymphaea lotus
Wintergreen	Gaultheria procumbens
Yarrow	Achillea millefolium
Ylang Ylang	Cananga odorata

Proven Benefits of Essential Oils

Now that you have the list of essential oils, you need to take some time to read about the many benefits and uses of these important tools. Essential oils have so many specific benefits to people of all ages, but particularly senior citizens. There are at least four general benefits when utilizing aromatherapy. These significant wellness effects are your key to a better quality of life in your senior years. First, essential oils ensure a cleaner environment. Second, they are responsible for improved physical well-being of many individuals particularly seniors. Third, these oils have been proven to aid mental clarity which is a major problem for those in their 60s and beyond. Fourth, essential oils boost emotional health as they provide a feeling of relief and can change negative moods to positive ones.

Aside from Dunst, the natural assistance available through aromatherapy is popular among such celebrities as Glenn Close, Brad Pitt, and Jennifer Aniston. What do they get from this traditional healing method? These celebrities and many other people, including elderly members of the family, enjoy benefits as enumerated below:

Healthier Environment. Some essential oils, when used in aromatherapy, make the environment cleaner. This is good news to the elderly! Because of their susceptibility to infections and other forms of illnesses, older people cannot afford living in unclean surroundings. With aromatherapy solutions and the of essential oils therein containing anti-bacterial and antiseptic properties, seniors can be assured of a healthier environment.

Improved Physical Well-Being. Aromatherapy or the use of essential oils has tremendous positive effects on the overall well-being of the body. This method of therapy has been proven to help improve one's immune system which is necessary to fight sicknesses. For elderly who have difficulty breathing, use of essential oils will help them breathe properly. Aromatherapy also helps boost energy levels, aids in digestion, and helps in cell regeneration by reducing or controlling wrinkles and skin discoloration. In addition, essential oils help relieve body aches and pains such as arthritis.

Increased Mental Clarity. One of the greatest benefits of aromatherapy is that it aids in achieving an overall mental clarity. The ability to focus and do what one needs to do at a given time is crucial especially for the elderly. Good thing, then, that there is aromatherapy available to help in a number of ways. As aging causes the loss of brain cells every day, memory loss is the eventual result. Aromatherapy helps improve memory which is a common aging problem. It is also responsible for increased cognitive performance.

Improved Emotional Health. Aside from achieving better physical and mental health, individuals engaged in aromatherapy find that their emotional state also improves, thanks to the helpful essential oils used. One of the most important healing effects of essential oils is their power to lift a person's mood due to their shooting properties. People who are depressed have been helped by using aromatherapy, finding comfort from a combination of essential oils. Aroma therapists also attest to the power of essential oils to enhance feelings of happiness. At the same time, overly anxious seniors can experience calmness through aromatherapy.

Just a reminder for those planning to use aromatherapy: Any forms of healing, whether the modern or the traditional way, can have some side effects and so it is important that you read the labels of available blends of essential oils. It is also better to seek medical advice, just to be sure prior to using aromatherapy, particularly from people knowledgeable on the subject such as health practitioners who are into integrative medicine, holistic health, or natural medicine.

Chapter 3- Why Every Home Should Have Essential Oils

Aromatherapy guru Geraldine Howard has found using essential oils to be of significant help in her post-cancer recovery (O'Brien, 2013). According to a report by the Daily Mail online, Howard made use of her own concoctions to deal with the blues induced by the post-operation procedures due to her eye cancer. For example, the UK-based aroma therapist used frankincense, cardamom, rosemary, sage, geranium, vetiver and sandalwood to address her problems ranging from lack of mental alertness, anxiety and stress issues, poor circulation, and digestion impairments brought about from the post-cancer state.

Many people, particularly the elderly are vulnerable to so many sicknesses and illnesses. The reason is that their immune system is weaker compared to others. The usual remedy is the use of maintenance drugs and vitamins from big pharmaceutical companies. There is, however, a natural way to deal with several aging-related concerns – from physical problems to emotional issues – by using essential oils. Essential oils are gifts to us. They are the answers to various illnesses associated with aging. In this chapter, I have provided a list of illnesses and which essential oils can be used for their amelioration. You will learn why every household should have essential oils.

Alzheimer's and Dementia. With old age, sicknesses like Alzheimer's and Dementia come uninvited. Essential oils help alleviate these sicknesses and their symptoms, partly by working to enhance memory among the elderly. Studies show that **rosemary, lemon, peppermint and basil** are effective in improving alertness. Inhaling the scent of the oils and a massage using a few drops can also aid in memory function.

Anxiety. Those living alone or in home care centers are often anxious about many things, primarily because they are not with family and can feel isolated. Citrus-based essential oils such as **orange** and **lemon** are proven to be effective in treating symptoms of anxiety. **Grapefruit, bergamot,** and **neroli** can also be used for this purpose. People who suffer from panic attacks can be administered with the Essential Oil of rose. **Peppermint** essential oil can also be used for anxiety-related problems.

Arthritis and Muscle Pains. Pains can be unbearable. Arthritis is paralyzing due to the pain caused by inflammation. Some people can't walk well and cry through the night because of arthritis. You can help your elderly family members with this problem by using essential oils from **rosemary, marjoram, veviter,** and **ginger.**

Marjoram, sandalwood, and **roman chamomile** have the same effects. Fluid build-up in the joints, common among the aging, can be treated with essential oils from **juniper berry.**

Blood Circulation. Because of inactivity and lack of exercise, the elderly have to deal with poor circulation. Using essential oils of **black pepper** or **peppermint** can help improve circulation. **Eucalyptus** is also proven to be effective in improving blood circulation.

Breathing Problems. The elderly also experience respiratory complications. Those involved in aromatherapy utilizing the appropriate essential oils find that they are greatly aided by certain oils to breathe well. Seniors can use **peppermint, clove, eucalyptus,** among others, for relief in breathing. For asthma for example, **chamomile, oregano, lavender, tea tree,** and **frankincense,** are effective remedies.

Calming and Sedative Effects. There are essential oils that are of big help because they give a relaxed feeling. When one is relaxed, they are able to function better. If they have the tendency to be restless, then they are best aided by the use of such essential oils as **lavender, clary sage (used in lower quantities),** and **ylang ylang**. These oils, aside from having calming effects, also lower blood pressure. If individuals are struggling with their sleep, the calming effects of oils will enable them to hit the sack when it's time to bed.

Depression. Depression is a common problem among the elderly. Like other people, they suffer from high cortisol levels which cause stress and depression. To decrease cortisol, essential oil from **rosemary** can be used. Other essential oils that can be helpful are those from **peppermint,** which boosts the mood and makes a person feel happy, and from **rose,** which is known to contain anti-depressant properties.

Digestive Problems. Some bodily functions are slowed due to aging. Giving our elderly loved ones some aromatherapy can help regulate their digestive tract. Essential oils of **marjoram, chamomile,** and **ginger** can be rubbed upon the abdominal area to relieve digestion problems. **Peppermint** is also known to help regulate our digestive tract

Headaches and Sinusitis. If your aging loved one is suffering from headaches, you can use **eucalyptus** and rosemary essential oils. Make these readily available at home for quick relief when discomfort strikes. **Eucalyptus** is also effective in treating sinus problems.

High Blood Pressure. Our elderly also deal with hypertension for a number of reasons such as lack of mobility and circulation problems. To help them, we can administer drops of essential oils for aromatherapy and these oils include **ylang**

ylang, **lavender**, and **clary sage**. These oils, aside from having calming effects, also lower blood pressure.

Inflammation. Inflammation can be treated with essential oils, and the good news is, there are several essential oils that have anti-inflammatory properties. These include **rosemary, juniper, peppermint, eucalyptus, sweet marjoram, frankincense, lavender, thyme, ginger, and wintergreen.**

Insomnia. The elderly wake up so early and they often sleep late. Worse, they are unable to fall asleep at all due to a number of reasons such as stress, anxiety, depression, and physical pains. You can help your aging loved one with the use of **peppermint** which has soothing properties for a majority of the aforementioned ailments. **Lavender**, too, helps them fall asleep due to its sedative effects. **Rosemary ylang ylang**, and **clary sage** also have calming effects and are effective in treating insomnia especially among seniors. Using them may help your elderly loved ones feel relaxed.

Lack of Energy. Weakness is a common problem among the elderly. Taking pills and supplements may help us cope, but don't you know that aromatherapy can achieve the same thing? One great benefit of essential oils is that they help improve energy levels and these include the essential oils of **peppermint**, among a few others. If you are fatigue and lethargic, it's time you tried this method!

Memory Loss. Some illnesses like Parkinson's disease, dementia, and Alzheimer's result in memory loss, which happens in many elderly people. Help them regain or enhance memory by using essential oils of **basil, lemon, rosemary**, and **peppermint**. The scent of these oils improves their mental alertness.

No Motivation. It is normal for your elderly loved ones to be sad or simply lacking the mood to move, talk or socialize. It is an emotional condition brought about by aging. To help them, use a drop of peppermint essential oil on a cotton ball. Place the cotton ball in an area near the person so he or she can smell the scent. That will give them the kick they need.

Respiratory Infections. Seniors are susceptible to common colds and coughs. They can also develop flu and acquire pneumonia due to their weak immune system. You can help your elderly loved ones by using essential oils of **peppermint, lavender, thyme**, and **eucalyptus smithii**. Other equally effective oils are those of **ravensara, rosemary**, and **tea trea**.

Scrapes and Cuts Disinfectant. The elderly, due to weakness and frailty, are vulnerable to falls, which at times become the cause of scrapes and cuts. First aid kits and medicines help, but there is actually a natural remedy. Some essential oils, like **chamomile, lavender,** and **tea tree,** have antibacterial properties, and as such they are very useful in treating minor cuts and scrapes. They also help control inflammation. **Rose,** which contains a compound known as farnesol, can help eliminate bacteria surrounding scrapes and cuts.

Softer Skin. Because the elderly can have cracked and dry skin, it will serve them well if we massage their bodies using a blend of unscented lotion and some essential oils. One option is to mix **peppermint** with a hypoallergenic lotion and use it to massage the body. Other great essential oils to blend with lotion are **citrus** and **lavender.**

Stimulate Appetite. If your loved one refuses to eat or barely touches his or her food, use an effective remedy. Before each meal, diffuse the scent of bergamot or ginger oil, cardamom, and citrus bliss in a place where the person lives. You may also use a cotton swab with drops of these oils and dab the swabs on their clothes at mealtime. Make sure you dab the part of the clothing close to the nose such as the collar, shoulder area, or the neck.

Stress. One problem associated with aging is stress. From one sickness to another, the elderly suffer from high levels of stress. They also get stressed from a number of other factors such as immobility, body pains, etc. With the use of essential oils like **veviter, bergamot, lavender, rose, chamomile, lemon, frankincense, cinnamon, geranium, rosewood** and **ylang ylang,** stress levels go down or are relieved completely.

Weak Immune System. As people age, their immune system weakens. This is due to a number of factors such as decreased food intake and circulation issues, among others. When this happens, they are more prone to diseases and bacterial and viral infections. This means, they get sick more easily because of increased susceptibility to infections. However, with the use of appropriate essential oils such as **tea tree, lemon, lavender, sandalwood, peppermint, bergamot, myrrh, thyme, Roman chamomile,** aging individuals are able to boost their immune system. Some essential oils help the body grow white blood cells that are essential in fighting illnesses.

Wrinkles and Discoloration. Aromatherapy using certain oils can actually help promote growth of cells in the body. This is good news for the elderly who have problems with their skin such as wrinkles. Some oils such as **rose, rosemary**, and **frankincense,** are proven effective to soften lines and improve complexion. **Carrot** is also used for the same purpose. These oils have antioxidants that help in boosting skin health.

Chapter 4- Preparing Special Blends of Essential Oils for Wellness

Essential oils can be combined for specific purposes such as treatment for certain conditions. In this chapter, I have provided you with certain blends for you to use for your elder-care. You can be confident that these blends can achieve the wellness you desire for your loved ones.

Understanding Carrier Oils

Blending essentials usually requires carrier oils. Also known as base oils, carrier oils are unscented and their function is for dilution. As many essential oils are highly concentrated and/or are strong, mixing them with base oils allows proper use for massages, inhalation, and baths.

Carrier or base oils commonly used for essential oil blends include the following: almond oil (sweet), aloe vera macerated oil, apricot kernel base oil, avocado crude oil, calendula macerated base oil, evening primrose base oil, grape seed oil, hazelnut base oil, jojoba oil, olive oil, macadamia nut oil, sesame seed oil, and wheatgerm oil.

Guidelines for Combining Essential Oils

Dilution Rate for Older People. There are certain specifications when combining essential oils with other oils. In the case of the elderly, it is important to use lower dilution rate for blends. As I have already stated, older people have sensitive skin and usually weaker. For people 65 years old and above, it is recommended that for every 20 ml of carrier oil, 5 drops of essential oil must be used. For people younger, drops are recommended. You can use the same blends for baths.

Strong Oils. Be sure you are familiar with oils that can cause irritations to older people. As stated in previous chapters, citrus-based oils as well as peppermints and eucalyptus are normally stronger and can cause irritations to sensitive skin.

How to Prepare Essential Oils Blends

Alternative Stress Blend. This is another blend for reducing stress. Combine the following: 5 drops of cistus essential oil, 30 drops of lavender, 20 drops of roman chamomile, and 10 drops of tangerine. Use as a massage oil or for inhalation. This can also be mixed with water during a bath.

Antiseptic Blend. A blend of essential oils used as an antiseptic is a must-have at home. You can prepare this on your own by combining the following: 15 drops of lavender essential oil, 20 drops of melaleuca, 20 drops of naouli, and 10 drops of rosemary.

Antiviral Blend. This can be prepared by combining the following: 8 drops of clove essential oil, 12 drops of peppermint, 8 drops of ravensara, 20 drops of sandalwood, 8 drops of tsuga, and 8 drops of thyme. This is a natural antiviral blend that your elderly must use.

Anxiety, Depression and Stress. To relieve anxiety, depression, and stress, a few drops of lavender can be used to massage the back of the neck along the spine. The elderly will immediately feel the effect of the essential oil as it penetrates the skin through which the brain picks ups signals that result in a relaxed feeling. To achieve happy emotions, you may try to prepare this recipe: sandalwood, spikenard, cedar, and patchouli mixed with golden jojoba bean liquid wax and grape seed oil. This blend is used for achieving positive or happy feelings and ideal for people who are restless, anxious, depressed, and unable to sleep.

Arthritis Blend. Combine 3 drops of roman chamomile, 3 drops of lavender, and 3 drops of lemon, and mix with 12 ml of your carrier oil such as sweet almond. This provides relief to the aching joints causes by arthritis. Make this available all the time for instant relief of your suffering elderly loved one.

Circulation Blend

Circulation is a major problem for many elderly. Here's a mixture that can be made and used with ease. Combine 10 drops of cypress essential oil, 24 drops of goldenrod, 8 drops of marjoram, and 4 drops of ylang ylang. Use as a massage oil or for inhalation. This can also be mixed with water during bath.

Clarity of Mind Recipe

Seniors usually have problems concentrating or paying attention. That comes with aging and family members have to live with that reality. Help your aging family member with this clarity blend. To prepare this blend, combine 40 drops of cardamom, 5 drops of peppermint, 30 drops of rosemary, and 10 drops of veviter. Use as a massage oil or for inhalation.

Cracked Skin

Our elderly also deal with skin issues. Due to circulation and hydration problems, their skin tends to crack due to dryness. You can help them by preparing this special blend, which can be used from time to time for skin hydration. To prepare this blend, combine 3 drops of lavender with your carrier oil of about 12 ml. Use it as a massage oil on affected skin.

Digestive Problems

Help your aging loved ones deal with their digestion problems. You can make your own blend of essential oils for relief of their digestive problems. Here's what you can do: Combine 30 drops of anise essential oil, 3 drops of blue tansy oil, 8 drops of fennel oil, 8 drops ginger, 25 rosemary oil, and 10 tarragon. Use as a rub on the abdomen area for digestion problems.

Energy Blend

Lack of energy is common among the aging population. Help them feel stronger and more vital with this energy blend. To make your elderly loved one feel energized, you can use this blend from time to time. Combine 30 drops of balsam fir essential oil, 25 drops of geraium, 20 drops of German chamomile, 20 drops of juniper, 10 drops of ledum, 10 drops of nutmeg, 40 drops of rosemary, 15 drops of sandalwood, and 30 drops of ylang ylang. Inhale the fragrance by putting a few drops on strips of paper. Use it also as a massage oil.

Essential Brain Blend

To awaken the brain and memory, use this blend. Combine 30 drops of balsam fir essential oil, 8 drops of helichrysm oil, 15 drops of frankincense, 3 drops of melissa, and 15 drops of sandalwood. Use as a massage oil or for inhalation.

Happiness Blend or Mood Lifters

It is always be a joy to see our elderly loved ones smiling. This happiness blend is a proven remedy to keep them cheerful and grinning. Simply mix the following ingredients: 1 drop of bergamot, 3 drops of clary sage, 3 drops of lavender, 4 drops of tangerine, 1 drop of ylang ylang III, and blend it with 1 teaspoon of FCO or fractionated coconut oil.

This can be stored in a roller bottle and applied like a perfume. This blend can also be used to relax the elderly and make them fall asleep.

Happiness through Inhaling To lift up the spirits of our

elderly, we can use essential oil of sweet orange and other anti-depression oils listed in Chapter 3. Put a few drops on fragrance strips and have them inhale the scent. You will notice that the fragrance will immediately make them feel good as you see them lighten up and smile. Be sure not to apply orange oil onto the skin without diluting it with base oils. You may also want to use a diffuser to achieve a relaxing mood around the house.

Headache Recipe Our elderly look to us for compassionate care. To

make them feel loved, we do all we can to attend to them. To relieve their headaches, for example, use this special blend of essential oils. It is easy to make. Simply combine 10 drops of basil, 3 drops of helichrysm, 8 drops of marjoram, and 10 drops of peppermint. Use as a massage oil on the temple and forehead.

High Blood Blend For elderly with bouts with high blood pressure,

this is welcome news. To prepare, just combine the following: 5 drops of cypress essential oil, 5 drops of marjoram, 10 drops of ylang ylang, and 1 oz. of any carrier oil. Use this as a massage oil. Apply on the chest area close to where the heart is. It can also be used when doing reflexology for your elderly, paying particular attention to the left foot and the hand.

Immune Booster Blend To ensure that our elderly loved ones are

protected from illnesses or at least they are less susceptible to infections, make use of this immune blend. This is how to prepare it: All you have to do is combine 5 drops of cumin, 20 drops of lemon, 30 mt. Savory, 5 drops of oregano, 20 drops of ravensa, 5 drops of tansy, and 10 drops of thyme.

Intestinal Ailments Combine 1 drop of chamomile, a drop of clove,

1 drop of peppermint, 2 drops of rosemary and blend them with 5 ml of any vegetable carrier oil available in the market. Use this blend as a massage oil on the belly especially where there is discomfort. Your elderly loved one will appreciate you for such relief.

Muscle Relief Blend. Be there for your aging member of the family

by helping them experience relief from muscle aches and pains. Prepare this muscle relief blend and voila! You have an instant treatment for them. This is easy to prepare. Make sure you have the following: 25 drops of balsam fir, 15 drops of basil, 10 drops of marjoram, 8 drops of spruce, and 4 drops of wintergreen. Combine all of these and you have a massage blend for aching muscles. Use as a massage oil to find relief from muscle aches and pains. The elderly will surely keep asking for this oil time and time again!

Nervous Tension.
Aging people experience nervous tensions for a number of reasons. It may be due to a current sickness or illness they are dealing with, loss of a loved one, and other aging-related concerns that can agitate them. Help your elderly experience calmness by preparing and using this blend. To prepare this recipe, combine 3 drops of lavender, 3 drops of mandarin, and 3 drops of orange.

Other Insomnia Blend.
Combine 5 drops of bergamot, 5 drops of clary sage, and 10 drops of roman chamomile. Use 1 or 2 drops of this mixture and apply on a tissue paper. Place the tissue under the pillow of your insomniac elderly and they will doze off in no time. You can also use this by putting 1 drop of bergamot, 1 drop of clary sage, 2 drops of roman chamomile. Alternatively, you can use 20 drops of lavender to 7 drops of vetiver. Put the blend in a roller bottle and add FCO or any other base oil, then roll on the feet of the person before they go to bed.

Pain Relief Recipe.
To prepare this recipe, mix 30 drops of balsam fir, 10 drops of helichrysm, 1 drop of oregano, and 5 drops of peppermint. Use as a massage oil for relief of pain. Your elderly loved one will appreciate you for this blend.

Perk up Effects.
To awaken your elderly, use rosemary, which enhances memory as discussed in the previous chapter. Put a few drops on strips of paper and have your elderly inhale the fragrance. This makes them alert and improved short and long-term memory!

Respiratory Problems.
Your elderly deal with respiratory complications from time to time. Give them this blend via massage or inhalation. To prepare this blend, combine 10 drops of cypress essential oil, 20 drops of eucalyptus australiana, 25 drops of eucalyptus radiata, 16 drops of myrtle, 5 drops of peppermint, 18 drops of ponderosa pine, and 30 drops of ravensara.

Trauma Blend.
Combine the following: 12 drops of cedarwood, 20 drops of davana, 15 drops of frankincense, 20 drops of kafir lime, 16 drops of lavender, 10 drops of spruce, 5 drops of rose, and 6 drops of tsuga. Use for massage or inhalation.

MRH Four Thieves Blends

One of the most popular and widely used blends of essential oils is that of MRH Four Thieves. MRH stands for Mountain Rose Herbs. MRH Four Thieves is useful in treating many conditions, which will be provided in this chapter.

Here's how to prepare this mixture: Combine 35 drops of cinnamon bark essential oil, 40 drops of clove bud essential oil, 15 drops of eucalyptus, 35 drops of lemon oil, and 10 drops of rosemary. Use dark-colored bottles for your mixture. When using this strong formula, make sure you dilute it first with the carrier oils. When diluting, use only between 1 to 2 % of this mixture with your base oil, meaning only between 6 to 12 drops of MRH are needed to combine with your carrier oil.

Nose Congestion. Combine a 1-2% dilution rate of MRH Four Thieves with jojoba or olive oil and rub under the nose or upon the chest area. To inhale, you can use two drops in a steaming bowl of water and let the person inhale the vapor under a towel. This will relieve nose congestion in no time.

Pain, Colds, and Flu. To find relief from aching muscles, make your own blend by mixing MRH Four Thieves with the carrier oil jojoba or olive oil. Dilution rate should be 1 to 2 % only. Use the mixture to massage aching muscles such as the feet, neck, and lower back. This blend is also used to strengthen the immune system and prevent colds and flu. All you do is dab the oil on the skin and use throughout the day.

Skin Problems. You can help your elderly find relief from their inflammation, skin irritation and itching with the use of MRH Four Thieves blended with other oils. Combine 1-2% dilution rate of MRH Four Thieves in a base of water or alcohol and store in a spray bottle. Spray on rashes and insect bites to reduce inflammation, itching, as well as irritation.

Citrus MRH Blend

You can have another form of MRH which is mostly citrus in content. Combine 1 drop of clary sage essential oil, 2 drops of lavender, 3 drops of lemon essential oil, 3 drops of lime, 3 drops orange oil, 1 drop nutmeg and 2 oz of witch hazel extract. Mix the oils in a 2 oz bottle with a mister top. This is ideal for spraying in homes for the elderly. It can also be used as a cleaning agent, the scent of which may be enjoyed by the aging.

Conclusion- Achieving a Better Life and Wellness Through Essential Oils

You can achieve a better, healthier life through natural means. And this is through the use of essential oils which are abundant, prevalent and on the rise in the current state of our culture. Essential oils are inexpensive and relatively easy to obtain. In addition, special blends, as discussed in Chapter 4, can easily be prepared and used by your elderly loved ones. Be sure to follow the preparation tips, especially the dilution rate information, for each essential oil. Remember, too, to ask your aging family members if they are comfortable with the scents you're planning to use for diffusers, candles, baths, or massages. They are, in the first place, the recipients of the therapy and it's important to ask their opinions as much as possible to ensure the highest quality of experience!

Use various essential oils as blends or as a stand-alone oil for various purposes, one such purpose being to disinfect your surroundings to protect your beloved elders from bacteria and viruses. Make the oils handy so you can use them regularly and with ease of access for massages to provide instant relief of cold symptoms, headaches, muscle pains, arthritis, and more. Give these blends as gifts as you try to help loved ones overcome stress and emotional and mental problems like anxiety, depression, nervous tension, and the like.

By a fraction of what is spent for unnatural conventional medicine, you allow your loved ones to have a greater quality life and experience wellness to the highest degree even in their sunset years. Using essential oils is also easy and side effects are minimal, if any.

You can at any time go through the information in this book so you are guided properly. Feel free to recommend it to your friends who are also involved with caring for the elderly. You will be glad you did. This is a very special gift that has the potential to restore optimal health and wellness for anyone in need, and I hope it finds you well.

-- *Yvonne Brooks*

For millions around the globe, care-giving is the "new normal" as the population continues to age.

Holistic symptom management for the elderly is an ever-increasing focus for medical and professional care facilities.

What if you could help your beloved elderly relax, calm down , treat symptoms of illnesses without the use of conventional medicines and tolerate their unpleasant side effects?

In this practical guide, you will learn about **Aroma-Care**. The use of Aromatherapy; an ancient alternative healing practice for improving overall health not only for your beloved elderly, but the entire family.
There is a long history of empirical evidence supporting the use of Aromatherapy as a preventive first line treatment for dementia and also to address symptoms such as sun downing, memory loss and sleep problems. There are many ways to receive Aromatherapy such as massages, oils, candles, baths and showers.

Here are some of the essential oil blends you will be learning to prepare:

- Antiseptic Blend
- Antiviral Blend
- Arthritis Blend
- Circulation blend
- Digestive problems blend
- Happiness Blend
- High Blood Blend
- Immune Booster Blend
- Trauma Blend
- MRH Four Thieves Blend
- Much, Much, More…

The psychological and physical well-being of your loved one is priceless!!
 Grab a copy now and start providing comfort for your beloved elderly now!

ISBN 9781534671263

90000

9 781534 671263

IN THE YEAR 1972.

KERRY BUTTERS.